HERBAL BOOK OF LOST NATURAL REMEDIES

Holistic Alternative Medicinal Wellness Guide of Cures for Common Health Issues

Chad M. Garcia

Copyright © Chad M. Garcia 2023. All rights reserved.

Table of Contents

INTRODUCTION: PURPOSE OF THE BOOK

Welcome to a voyage through the rich tapestry of herbal remedies—a collection of old knowledge and lost therapies. This introduction serves as the entryway to a world where the therapeutic touch of nature intertwines with centuries-old traditions, bringing consolation and well-being to individuals seeking alternatives to contemporary medications.

Embarking on a Natural Odyssey: Delve into the goal of this book as a guide to unearthing the gems buried inside the plant world. Explore the core of herbalism as a holistic approach to health, connecting with the body's natural cycles.

Revitalizing Ancient Wisdom: Uncover the importance of conserving and revitalizing age-old herbal knowledge, sometimes on the verge of extinction. Reflect on the eternal potency of herbal treatments, reflecting the traditions of our ancestors.

A Call to Holistic Wellness: Illuminate the book's purpose to encourage readers to take ownership of their well-being via natural alternatives. Discuss the limits of traditional medicine and the possibilities of herbalism to enhance contemporary healthcare.

Connecting with Nature's Pharmacy: Paint a vivid image of the vast botanical world, showing the great healing potential found in plants. Encourage readers to establish a stronger relationship with nature, acknowledging it as the ultimate apothecary.

Navigating the Pages Ahead: Provide a quick summary of the subject divisions and chapters, offering readers a guide for their investigation. Tease the tempting assortment of missing treatments waiting to be revealed inside the next pages.

Igniting Curiosity and Inquiry: Pose thought-provoking questions to pique readers' curiosity about the holistic cosmos of herbal therapy. Invite thought on the interdependence of human health with the natural environment.

Setting the Tone: Establish a tone of regard for the ancient healing arts, fostering an environment of respect for the knowledge contained in traditional techniques. Convey the hope that this book will serve as a spark for a resurgence in herbalism.

As you begin on this herbal voyage, let the following pages guide you into the heart of forgotten remedies, where the whispers of the past resonate through the leaves and roots, giving a sanctuary of healing wisdom waiting to be unearthed.

BRIEF HISTORY OF HERBAL REMEDIES

Embark on a voyage through the annals of time as we explore the origins and development of herbal cures, revealing a tale woven into the very fabric of human life.

Ancient wisdom (3000 BCE - 500 CE): Explore the oldest records of herbal medicine in ancient civilizations, including Mesopotamia, Egypt, and China. Delve into the Ebers Papyrus and Shen Nong's Herbal Classic, key writings that set the foundations for herbal medicine.

Greece and Rome (500 BCE - 500 CE): Witness the rise of herbalism in the hands of famous characters like Hippocrates and Dioscorides. Uncover the herbal wisdom in mythology and ancient Greece's herbal gardens.

The Middle Ages (500 - 1500 CE): Navigate the medieval era, when monasteries were centers of herbal study and preservation. Encounter the significant work of herbalists like Hildegard von Bingen and the development of herbals, such as the Trotula.

Renaissance and Exploration (1400 - 1700 CE): Witness the return of interest in botanical sciences during the Renaissance. Explore the herbal voyages of exploration, bringing new plants and treatments from faraway regions to Europe.

The Age of Enlightenment (1700 - 1800 CE): Analyze the scientific breakthroughs impacting herbal medicine throughout the Enlightenment. Witness the publishing of major publications like Linnaeus's "Species Plantarum" and the standardization of botanical terminology.

19th Century and Modern Revival (1800 - Present): Examine the influence of industrialization on herbal therapy and the emergence of botanical pharmacology. Explore the Renaissance of interest in herbalism in the 20th century, characterized by the contributions of herbalists like Juliette de Bairacli Levy and Rosemary Gladstar.

Global Traditions and Indigenous Wisdom: Acknowledge the varied herbal traditions across the globe, from Ayurveda in India to the healing practices of Indigenous nations. Emphasize the necessity of conserving and appreciating traditional knowledge in a globalized society.

This trip through time shows the ongoing thread of herbal cures woven throughout human history—a monument to the lasting bond between humans and the therapeutic wealth of the plant world.

UNDERSTANDING HERBAL MEDICINE: PRINCIPLES OF HERBAL HEALING

Embark on a voyage of discovery as we explore the basic concepts that support the art and science of herbal medicine, building a link between humanity and the delicate dance of nature.

Holistic Harmony: Delve into the holistic approach of herbal medicine, acknowledging the interdependence of mind, body, and spirit. Explore how herbal treatments aim to restore balance and harmony, treating the fundamental causes of diseases.

Vital Energy and Herbalism: Uncover critical energy, known as qi in Traditional Chinese Medicine or prana in Ayurveda. Discuss how herbs are thought to impact and promote the flow of vital energy, supporting general well-being.

The Doctrine of Signatures: Examine the ancient notion that plants resemble the bodily parts they may treat, a concept known as the Doctrine of Signatures. Explore how this theory assisted herbalists in finding herbs for certain diseases.

Synergy of Plant substances: Investigate the synergistic interaction of substances inside plants, such as alkaloids, flavonoids, and essential oils. Understand how combining these substances adds to the therapeutic effectiveness of herbal treatments.

Adaptogenic Wisdom: Explore the adaptogenic characteristics of specific herbs, which help the body adapt to stress and preserve equilibrium. Discuss the significance of adaptogens in boosting the body's resilience and increasing general vitality.

Seasonal and Circadian cycles: Recognize the value of matching herbal treatments with seasonal and circadian cycles.

Understand how nature's cycles impact the potency and usefulness of certain plants throughout different seasons of the year.

Patient-Centered Care: Emphasize the customized aspect of herbal therapy, adapting medicines to each person's particular constitution and requirements. Discuss the significance of incorporating lifestyle, emotional well-being, and environmental aspects in herbal therapy.

By immersing ourselves in these principles, we open the door to a deeper knowledge of herbal medicine—a journey guided by the wisdom of nature and the delicate interaction of ingredients that contribute to our well-being.

IMPORTANCE OF PLANT IDENTIFICATION

Safety First: Emphasize the crucial significance of correct plant identification in guaranteeing the safety of herbal treatments. Highlight the hazards of misidentification and the need to differentiate between medicinal and dangerous plants.

Effectiveness and Potency: Discuss how exact identification assures the use of the proper plant species, enhancing the effectiveness and potency of herbal remedies. Explore the variances in chemical composition across various species, highlighting the necessity for precision.

Cultural and Traditional Values: Acknowledge distinct plant species' cultural and traditional values in diverse herbal therapies. Highlight the significance of conserving and honoring indigenous knowledge linked to plant identification.

Biodiversity Conservation: Stress the relationship between correct plant identification and biodiversity conservation. Explore the possible ecological effects of misidentifying or over-harvesting certain plant species.

Legal & Regulatory Compliance: Discuss the legal and regulatory considerations surrounding herbal medicine and the requirement for compliance with rules on plant identification. Highlight the ramifications of employing endangered or protected plant species.

Facilitating study and Education: Illustrate how exact plant identification promotes scientific study on herbal treatments. Discuss its importance in expanding our knowledge of plant chemistry, pharmacology, and medicinal uses.

Empowering Herbalists and Practitioners: Emphasize how correct plant identification helps herbalists and practitioners to identify and propose suitable medicines confidently. Discuss the relevance of continual education in remaining informed on botanical classifications and plant identification procedures.

Link to Nature: Explore the significant link between plant identification and cultivating a deeper relationship with the natural world. Encourage enthusiasts to participate in the art of plant identification as a method of building a deeper awareness of biodiversity.

By underlining the significance of plant identification, we assure the safe, effective, and sustainable application of nature's pharmacy, maintaining old knowledge while navigating the complicated and varied terrain of herbal medicine.

SUSTAINABLE HARVESTING PRACTICES

Respect for Nature's Rhythms: Emphasize the need to synchronize harvesting operations with natural cycles and seasons. Encourage practitioners to watch and respect the life cycles of plants, harvesting when their vitality is at its optimum.

Selective Harvesting: Advocate for selective harvesting to support the conservation of plant populations. Discuss the probable ecological consequences of over-harvesting and the significance of leaving enough plants for reproduction.

Ethical Wildcrafting: Introduce the notion of ethical wildcrafting, stressing the necessity for responsible and sustainable gathering in the wild. Highlight the effect of wildcrafting on biodiversity and the sensitive environments where these plants flourish.

Cultivation and Regeneration: Explore sustainable cultivation approaches, fostering the regeneration of medicinal plants. Discuss the advantages of farming at-risk species to ease the strain on wild populations.

Local and Indigenous Knowledge: Acknowledge the relevance of local and indigenous knowledge in sustainable harvesting. Encourage partnership with local people to learn from their traditional traditions and implement sustainable ways.

Harvesting practices: Guide correct harvesting practices to prevent harm to plants and ecosystems. Discuss the significance of employing instruments that allow for a clean cut, supporting plant health and regeneration.

Conservation relationships: Advocate for relationships with conservation groups to help preserve medicinal plant environments. Discuss the relevance of such cooperation in safeguarding the sustainability of herbal resources.

Education and Awareness: Stress the significance of educating herbalists, hobbyists, and the general public about sustainable harvesting. Highlight how increasing understanding may lead to more informed decisions and actions.

Legal Considerations: Discuss pertinent rules and regulations connected to the harvesting of medicinal plants. Emphasize the need to comply with legal requirements to safeguard plant populations and practitioners.

Quality above Quantity: Encourage a mentality that favors the quality of harvested plants over quantity. Discuss how a meticulous approach to harvesting leads to the strength and efficacy of herbal treatments.

By accepting these sustainable harvesting techniques, herbalists preserve biodiversity, the health of ecosystems, and the longevity of traditional herbal expertise, preserving a healthy interaction between humankind and the therapeutic gifts of the plant world.

HERBAL PREPARATION TECHNIQUES: INFUSIONS AND DECOCTIONS

Understanding the Basics: Introduce the essential distinction between infusions and decoctions. Highlight their mutual objective: obtaining therapeutic compounds from plants via water.

Herb Selection and Quality: Emphasize the necessity of choosing high-quality, dried herbs for maximum outcomes. Discuss factors for picking certain herbs based on their water-soluble components and medicinal effects.

Infusions Unveiled: Detail the method of preparing herbal infusions by steeping fragile plant pieces like leaves and petals. Explore this category's diversity of teas, tisanes, and medicinal infusions.

Decoctions Demystified: Illuminate the technique of preparing decoctions, often incorporating harder plant parts like roots, bark, and seeds. Discuss the simmering or boiling procedure to extract powerful components from hardy plant sections.

Proper Brewing Techniques: Provide step-by-step directions for making infusions and decoctions, guaranteeing optimum extraction.

Discuss temperature, steeping durations, and ratios to produce the appropriate strength and taste.

Choosing the Right Vessels: Guide readers on picking acceptable vessels for brewing, considering materials that won't damage the medicinal characteristics of the plants. Discuss the advantages of utilizing glass, ceramic, or stainless-steel containers.

Straining and Storing: Emphasize the need for straining herbal infusions and decoctions to eliminate plant debris. Provide recommendations on optimal storage to retain freshness and potency.

Enhancing Flavor and Efficacy: Explore innovative methods to increase the flavor of infusions, such as adding herbs, spices, or natural sweeteners. Discuss strategies to maximize the effectiveness of infusions, such as allowing particular herbs to soak longer for greater potency.

Customizing for Health Goals: Encourage readers to create infusions and decoctions based on specific health requirements. Provide instances of herbs good for diverse health aims, such as relaxation, immunological support, or digestive help.

Exploring Beyond the Cup: Inspire creativity by presenting alternate uses for herbal infusions and decoctions, such as integrating them into recipes or utilizing them for topical purposes.

By learning the art of herbal infusions and decoctions, readers start on a journey to uncover the healing power inside plants, converting simple rituals of brewing into profound acts of self-care and well-being.

TINCTURES AND EXTRACTS

Essence of Concentration: Introduce tinctures and extracts as concentrated herbal remedies meant to capture the essence of plant ingredients. Highlight their efficacy and adaptability in providing therapeutic effects.

Choosing the Right Solvent: Discuss the selection of acceptable solvents, often alcohol or glycerin, for extracting and preserving therapeutic ingredients. Explore the benefits and downsides of alternative solvents, considering alcohol's effectiveness in extracting a wide range of chemicals.

Understanding Ratios: Explain the need to maintain appropriate herb-to-solvent ratios for efficient extraction. Discuss how varied ratios affect the strength and potency of the final tincture or extract.

Herb Selection and Quality: Emphasize the need to utilize high-quality, dried herbs for tincture and extract preparations. Discuss factors for picking herbs based on their solubility in various solvents.

Conventional vs. Folk procedures: Contrast conventional maceration procedures with folk methods like percolation or the folklore "simpler's" approach. Discuss the merits and subtleties of each approach in terms of extraction efficiency.

Extraction length and Techniques: Guide readers on establishing the ideal extraction length, considering parameters such as herb kind and desired strength. Introduce strategies like twofold extraction for increasing the extraction of water-soluble and alcohol-soluble chemicals.

Straining and Filtration: Emphasize the need for thorough straining and filtration to eliminate plant debris and guarantee clarity. Discuss strategies to produce a clean, visually pleasing tincture or extract.

Dose and Administration: Provide guidelines on establishing suitable dose levels for tinctures and extracts. Discuss numerous delivery routes, such as sublingual, topical, or diluted liquids.

Alcohol-Free Alternatives: Cater to various tastes by researching alcohol-free alternatives such as glycerites or vinegar-based extracts. Discuss their applications and implications for individuals avoiding alcohol.

Storage and Shelf Life: Educate readers on correct storage conditions to ensure the life of tinctures and extracts. Discuss variables affecting shelf life and strategies to spot indicators of degradation.

By diving into the art of producing tinctures and extracts, readers discover the alchemical synergy between herbs and solvents, converting nature's gift into strong elixirs embodying the plant world's healing spirit.

POULTICES AND COMPRESSES

Introduction to External Herbal Applications: Introduce the notion of poultices and compresses as external applications for harnessing the medicinal powers of herbs. Highlight their adaptability in managing localized problems and fostering external recovery.

Poultices: Poultices are soft, wet things applied to the skin, generally containing crushed or mashed herbs. Discuss the advantages of poultices in giving direct herbal effects to particular body parts.

Compresses: Explain compresses as cloth or bandages soaked in herbal infusions or decoctions and applied to the skin. Explore compresses for both hot and cold treatments, depending on therapeutic aims.

Selecting Herbs for External Use: Emphasize the significance of picking herbs with particular qualities appropriate for external uses. Discuss plants recognized for their anti-inflammatory, analgesic, or antibacterial actions.

Preparation Techniques: Guide readers through the stages of creating poultices, stressing correct herb preparation and consistency. Discuss strategies for preparing herbal compresses, including hot and cold versions.

Application Methods: Provide instructions on applying poultices directly to the skin and fastening them with bandages or fabric. Discuss several procedures for applying compresses, including soaking, wringing, and layering.

Heated and Cold Therapies: Explore the advantages of heated poultices or compresses for easing muscular tension and promoting circulation. Discuss the benefits of cold treatments in lowering inflammation and relieving pain.

Targeted Healing: Highlight particular applications of poultices and compresses for ailments such as bruises, sprains, bug bites, or joint discomfort. Encourage readers to personalize herbal selections depending on the intended therapeutic benefits.

Safety Considerations: Address safety concerns, such as evaluating herbal temperatures before application and confirming skin compatibility. Discuss possible allergic responses and the significance of speaking with a healthcare expert for specific situations.

Incorporating Aromatherapy: Explore the added advantages of aromatherapy while utilizing herbs in poultices and compresses. Discuss how the aromatic characteristics of herbs contribute to a holistic healing experience.

By mastering the skill of poultices and compresses, readers uncover the possibility of focused external healing, establishing a stronger connection between herbs and the body's intrinsic capacity to restore balance and well-being.

COMMON AILMENTS AND CORRESPONDING REMEDIES: RESPIRATORY SYSTEM

Introduction to Respiratory Health: Highlight the critical function of the respiratory system in general well-being. Introduce the notion of employing herbal treatments to enhance respiratory health

Coughs & Congestion: Discuss herbs recognized for their expectorant characteristics to ease coughs and remove respiratory congestion. For powerful alleviation, explore medicines such as thyme, eucalyptus, and licorice root.

Bronchial Health: Introduce herbs that promote bronchial health and alleviate inflammation. Discuss the advantages of plants, including mullein, marshmallow root, and elecampane, in enhancing respiratory comfort.

Immune-Boosting Elixirs: Explore herbs famous for their immune-boosting capabilities to avoid respiratory infections. Discuss remedies utilizing echinacea, elderberry, and astragalus to reinforce the body's defenses.

Allergy Relief: Discuss herbal approaches for reducing respiratory allergies and hay fever symptoms. Explore the usage of nettles, butterbur, and quercetin-rich plants for natural allergy support.

Asthma Support: Address herbal choices for controlling asthma symptoms and enhancing respiratory relaxation. Discuss the role of herbs like boswellia, lobelia, and ginger in promoting respiratory function.

Lung-cleaning Teas: Introduce herbal teas particularly created for cleaning and strengthening the lungs. Explore combinations incorporating lung-friendly herbs like fenugreek, oregano, and peppermint.

Steam Inhalations: Discuss the usage of steam inhalations with respiratory-friendly herbs. Explore the advantages of breathing vapor from herbs like eucalyptus, chamomile, and Rosemary for respiratory comfort.

Creating Herbal Syrups: Guide readers in producing herbal syrups to soothe and coat the respiratory tract. Discuss recipes incorporating herbs such as honey, thyme, and marshmallow root for their calming effects.

Preventive choices: Emphasize lifestyle and nutritional choices that contribute to respiratory health. Discuss the significance of drinking, having a clean environment, and including respiratory-friendly foods in the diet.

By researching these herbal treatments for the respiratory system, readers may nurture lung health, relieve common respiratory disorders, and proactively support the body's capacity to breathe comfortably.

HERBAL SYRUPS FOR COUGH

Introduction to Herbal Syrups: Highlight the usefulness of herbal syrups as a pleasant and appealing approach to give therapeutic plants. Introduce the notion of utilizing syrups as a calming cure for coughs.

Honey as a basis: Discuss the advantages of utilizing raw honey as a basis for herbal syrups. Highlight honey's inherent antibacterial and calming effects on the respiratory tract.

Key plants for Cough Relief: Introduce plants famous for their cough-suppressant, expectorant, and relaxing characteristics. Discuss the utilization of thyme, licorice root, and marshmallow root for their distinct contributions.

Thyme Infused Syrup: Guide readers in producing a thyme-infused syrup for its robust antibacterial and expectorant effects. Discuss changes like adding lemon or ginger to boost taste and efficacy.

Licorice and Honey Blend: Explore the advantages of licorice root for healing inflamed throats and minimizing coughing. Provide a recipe for a licorice-infused honey syrup, showcasing its sweet and soothing qualities.

Marshmallow Root Soother: Discuss the mucilaginous characteristics of marshmallow root for coating and relaxing the respiratory system. Guide readers in creating a marshmallow root syrup with extra herbs for greater potency.

Ginger and Lemon Zest Elixir: Explore ginger's warming and immune-supportive qualities. Share a recipe for ginger and lemon zest syrup that calms coughs and promotes general respiratory health.

Elderberry Cough Syrup: Discuss the immune-boosting advantages of elderberry for cough alleviation. Provide a recipe for an elderberry-infused syrup, stressing its potential to decrease the duration of respiratory illnesses.

Dose and Administration: Educate readers on the proper dose depending on age and severity of symptoms. Discuss alternative administration strategies, such as ingesting the syrup straight or adding it to warm liquids.

Storage and Shelf Life: Guide readers on suitable storage procedures to retain the syrup's freshness and strength. Discuss the normal shelf life of herbal syrups and indicators of decomposition.

By preparing and adopting these herbal syrups into their health regimen, folks may enjoy the comforting embrace of natural medicines for cough alleviation, nurturing respiratory relaxation with the sweet healing touch of botanical elixirs.

LUNG-CLEANSING TEAS

Introduction to Lung-Cleaning Teas: Highlight the relevance of herbal teas in enhancing respiratory health and cleaning the lungs. Emphasize tea's natural, pleasant aspect as a delivery mechanism for lung-friendly herbs.

Eucalyptus and Peppermint Blend: Discuss eucalyptus and peppermint's decongestant and expectorant characteristics. Provide a pleasant tea mix recipe that helps cleanse the respiratory passages and soothe the throat.

Thyme and Sage Infusion: Explore thyme's antibacterial capabilities and sage's relaxing benefits on the respiratory system. Guide readers in brewing a thyme and sage tea to enhance respiratory health and relieve coughing.

Fenugreek and Fennel Soother: Discuss fenugreek's mucilaginous qualities and fennel's respiratory advantages. Provide a recipe for fenugreek and fennel tea that assists in mucus clearing and calms respiratory discomfort.

Oregano and Lemon Zest Elixir: Highlight oregano's antibacterial capabilities and the immune-boosting benefits of lemon zest. Share an oregano and lemon tea recipe that helps lung health and general respiratory well-being.

Licorice and Ginger Harmony: Explore licorice's relaxing effects and ginger's anti-inflammatory capabilities. Guide readers in brewing licorice and ginger tea to ease respiratory symptoms and improve immunological function.

Mullein and Marshmallow Root Infusion: Discuss the mucilaginous characteristics of mullein and marshmallow root for healing sore lungs. Provide a recipe for a mullein and marshmallow root tea that assists in respiratory health and comfort.

Nettle and Peppermint Detox Tea: Highlight nettle's cleansing powers and peppermint's pleasant features. Share a recipe for a nettle and peppermint tea that aids lung cleansing and delivers a refreshing feeling.

Rosemary and Lemon Balm Brew: Discuss the respiratory advantages of Rosemary and the relaxing effects of lemon balm. Provide a recipe for a rosemary and lemon balm tea that cleanses the lungs and encourages relaxation.

Introducing Tea into Daily Routine: Offer tips on introducing lung-cleansing drinks into daily activities. Discuss appropriate periods for tea drinking and other lifestyle alterations to boost respiratory well-being.

By drinking these lung-cleansing herbal teas, users may appreciate the therapeutic advantages of nature.

DIGESTIVE DISORDERS

Introduction to Herbal Support for Digestive Illness: Highlight the function of herbal medicines in maintaining digestive well-being and managing common illnesses. Emphasize the holistic approach of herbal treatment to assist the whole digestive system.

Peppermint and Chamomile Tea for Indigestion: Discuss peppermint's capacity to relieve digestive muscles and chamomile's soothing impact on the stomach. Provide a peppermint and chamomile tea recipe to reduce indigestion and encourage relaxation.

Ginger Infusion for Nausea: Explore ginger's anti-nausea characteristics and its usefulness in settling an upset stomach. Guide readers in brewing a ginger infusion to alleviate nausea and increase overall digestive comfort.

Fennel Seed Tea for Bloating: Discuss fennel seed's carminative characteristics, which help reduce gas and bloating. Provide a recipe for a fennel seed tea to relieve bloating and maintain a healthy digestive tract.

Dandelion and Burdock Root Detox Tea: Highlight dandelion and burdock root's potential to boost liver function and help in detoxification. Share a recipe for a dandelion and burdock root tea to maintain a healthy liver and digestive tract.

Licorice Root Elixir for Acid Reflux: Explore licorice root's relaxing effects on the digestive system and its ability to alleviate acid reflux. Guide readers in making a licorice root elixir to relieve acid reflux and enhance digestive relaxation.

Chamomile and Lemon Balm Blend for Stress-Induced Digestive Issues: Discuss the influence of stress on digestion and the relaxing characteristics of chamomile and lemon balm. Provide a chamomile and lemon balm tea recipe to treat stress-related stomach problems.

Minty Lemon Verbena Tea for IBS Relief: Explore the possible advantages of lemon verbena in controlling irritable bowel syndrome (IBS) symptoms. Share a recipe for a minty lemon verbena tea to reduce IBS-related pain and improve digestive equilibrium.

Gentle Aloe Vera Drink for Digestive Therapeutic: Discuss aloe vera's therapeutic benefits for the digestive system. Guide readers in creating a soothing aloe vera drink to help digestive healing and minimize inflammation.

Incorporating Herbal Bitters into Daily Routine: Discuss the advantages of herbal bitters in encouraging good digestion. Offer tips on adding herbal bitters into daily practices for continued digestive assistance.

By including these herbal medicines in their regimen, people may foster digestive harmony, ease pain, and promote the general well-being of their digestive system.

HERBAL BITTERS FOR INDIGESTION

Introduction to Herbal Bitters: Highlight the centuries-old history of utilizing bitters to assist digestion. Emphasize the importance of herbal bitters in activating digestive enzymes and enhancing overall digestive health.

Understanding Bitter Plants: Discuss the numerous bitter plants recognized for their digestive effects, such as gentian, dandelion, and artichoke. Explore the numerous components inside bitter plants that contribute to their potency.

Gentian Elixir for Digestive Stimulation: Introduce gentian as a powerful bitter herb recognized for boosting digestive processes. Provide a recipe for a gentian elixir that aids digestion and alleviates dyspepsia.

Dandelion and Burdock Infusion: Discuss dandelion and burdock as bitter herbs that help liver function and encourage detoxification. Share a recipe for a dandelion and burdock infusion, stressing its function in promoting overall digestive well-being.

Artichoke Leaf Tonic for Liver Support: Explore artichoke leaf's bitter components that improve liver and gallbladder function. Provide a recipe for an artichoke leaf tonic to boost bile production and aid digestion.

Fennel and Orange Bitter Elixir: Discuss fennel's carminative characteristics and the inclusion of orange for a nice taste. Guide readers in constructing a fennel and orange bitter elixir to alleviate indigestion and enhance digestive comfort.

Calendula and Chamomile Bitters for Soothing: Highlight calendula and chamomile's soft, soothing characteristics. Share a recipe for calendula and chamomile bitters for persons with delicate digestive systems.

Developing a unique Bitter Blend: Encourage readers to experiment with creating their special bitter mixes. Suggest balancing bitter, sweet, and aromatic herbs for a well-rounded and delicious taste.

Usage & Dosage Guidance: Discuss the ideal times for taking herbal bitters before meals to assist digestion. Offer advice on dose based on individual requirements.

SOOTHING TEAS FOR UPSET STOMACH

Introduction to Soothing Teas Highlights herbal teas' calming and therapeutic benefits for easing upset stomach. Emphasize the mild nature of herbal infusions in encouraging digestive relaxation.

Peppermint and Ginger Tisane: Discuss peppermint's relaxing effects on the digestive system and ginger's anti-nausea characteristics. Provide a peppermint and ginger tisane recipe to soothe an upset stomach and ease nausea.

Chamomile and Lemon Balm Infusion: Explore chamomile's anti-inflammatory benefits and lemon balm's relaxing effects. Share a chamomile and lemon balm infusion recipe to soothe the digestive tract and reduce pain.

Fennel and Cardamom Elixir: Discuss fennel's carminative characteristics and cardamom's potential to ease indigestion. Provide a fennel and cardamom elixir recipe to stimulate digestion and calm an upset stomach.

Licorice and Marshmallow Root Blend: Highlight licorice's relaxing virtues and marshmallow root's mucilaginous capabilities. Share a recipe for a licorice and marshmallow root tea combination to coat and quiet the digestive system.

Cinnamon and Banana Tea: Explore cinnamon's digestive advantages and the relaxing qualities of bananas. Provide a cinnamon and banana tea recipe to calm upset stomachs and add a touch of sweetness

Gentian and Lemon Verbena Tonic: Introduce gentian as a bitter herb for digestive stimulation and lemon verbena for taste. Guide readers in creating a gentian and lemon verbena tonic for light digestive help.

Chai-Inspired Minty Elixir: Combine peppermint's digestive benefits with chai spices' warmth. Share a recipe for a chai-inspired minty elixir to ease the stomach and bring comfort.

Lemon Ginger Soother: Discuss the digestive advantages of both lemon and ginger. Offer a lemon ginger tea recipe to reduce indigestion nausea and offer a pleasant taste.

Sipping Rituals for Digestive Ease: Encourage readers to use thoughtful sipping rituals while drinking calming teas. Share tips for establishing a relaxing setting to improve the overall therapeutic experience.

By sipping these calming herbal teas, folks may gradually relieve an upset stomach, promoting comfort and well-being.

SKIN CONDITIONS

Introduction to Herbal Skin Care: Highlight the comprehensive approach of herbal medicines in boosting skin health. Emphasize the significance of herbs in managing a range of skin disorders.

Calendula Salve for Irritated Skin: Discuss calendula's anti-inflammatory and healing capabilities. Share a recipe for a calendula salve to soothe and encourage the healing of sensitive skin.

Chamomile and Lavender Infused Oil for Eczema: Explore chamomile's anti-itch and anti-inflammatory benefits. Provide a recipe for chamomile and lavender-infused oil to treat symptoms of eczema.

Aloe Vera Gel and Tea Tree for Acne: Highlight tea tree oil's antibacterial qualities and aloe vera's calming benefits. Share a recipe for a tea tree and aloe vera gel to fight acne and decrease inflammation.

Oatmeal Bath for Dermatitis: Discuss the anti-inflammatory and calming effects of oatmeal. Provide a recipe for an oatmeal soak to treat dermatitis symptoms and soothe inflamed skin.

Comfrey Compress for Wound Healing: Explore comfrey's reputation for boosting tissue restoration. Share a comfrey compress recipe to help heal wounds and decrease inflammation.

Yarrow Tincture for Rosacea: Discuss Yarrow's anti-inflammatory capabilities. Provide a recipe for a yarrow tincture to assist in controlling symptoms of rosacea.

Licorice Root Serum for Hyperpigmentation: Highlight licorice root's skin-brightening effects. Share a recipe for a licorice root serum to reduce hyperpigmentation and even skin tone.

Witch Hazel Toner for Oily Skin: Explore witch hazel's astringent characteristics. Provide a witch hazel toner recipe to balance oily skin and minimize pore size.

Holistic Lifestyle Tips for Radiant Skin: Encourage holistic lifestyle habits for preserving healthy skin. Discuss the significance of hydration, a balanced diet, and stress management in maintaining overall skin well-being.

By adopting these herbal treatments and taking a holistic approach to skincare, people may nourish their skin, ease common ailments, and promote a beautiful and healthy complexion.

HERBAL SALVES FOR SKIN IRRITATIONS

Introduction to Herbal Salves: Emphasize the usefulness of herbal salves in topical treatment for different skin irritations. Highlight the natural therapeutic qualities of herbs in boosting skin well-being.

Calendula and Chamomile Soothing Salve: Discuss calendula's anti-inflammatory and chamomile's relaxing benefits. Share a recipe for a soothing ointment containing calendula and chamomile to treat skin irritations.

Lavender and Tea Tree Antiseptic Balm: Highlight lavender's calming effects and tea tree's antibacterial advantages. Provide a recipe for an antibacterial balm infused with lavender and tea tree to relieve skin irritations and aid healing.

Comfrey and Plantain Herbal Healing Ointment: Explore comfrey's tissue-healing capabilities and plantain's relaxing benefits. Share an herbal healing ointment recipe, including comfrey and plantain, to assist skin repair.

Arnica and St. John's Wort Pain Relief Salve: Discuss Arnica's anti-inflammatory characteristics and St. John's Wort's potential for pain relief. Provide a pain treatment ointment recipe using Arnica and St. John's Wort for soothing inflamed skin.

Yarrow and Calendula Wound Care Salve: Highlight Yarrow's antibacterial characteristics and calendula's wound-healing powers. Share a recipe for a wound care ointment using Yarrow and calendula to help heal.

Chickweed and Marshmallow Root Cooling Balm: Explore chickweed's cooling benefits and marshmallow root's mucilaginous characteristics. Provide a recipe for a cooling balm using chickweed and marshmallow root to alleviate heat-related skin irritations.

Plantain and Echinacea Anti-Itch Salve: Discuss plantain's anti-itch capabilities and echinacea's immune-supportive benefits. Share a recipe for an anti-itch salve with plantain and echinacea to ease itching and irritation.

Frankincense and Myrrh Skin Regeneration Salve: Highlight the skin-regenerating benefits of frankincense and myrrh. Provide a recipe for a skin regeneration salve containing frankincense and myrrh to boost general skin health.

Storage and Application Tips: Offer information on appropriate storage of herbal salves to ensure freshness and effectiveness. Discuss application methods, stressing the significance of clean hands and a delicate touch when applying salves to inflamed skin.

By preparing and using these herbal salves, people may harness nature's healing power to relieve different skin irritations, nurturing skin health and well-being.

ACNE-FIGHTING HERBAL MASKS

Introduction to Acne-Fighting Herbal Masks: Emphasize herbal masks' natural and holistic approach to controlling acne. Highlight the cleansing and relaxing characteristics of herbs for cleaner skin.

Tea Tree and Clay Detox Mask: Discuss tea tree oil's antibacterial characteristics and the oil-absorbing advantages of clay. Share a recipe for a tea tree and clay detox mask to cleanse pores and minimize acne-causing germs.

Turmeric and Honey Anti-Inflammatory Mask: Highlight turmeric's anti-inflammatory benefits and honey's antibacterial characteristics. Provide a turmeric and honey mask recipe to ease inflammation and promote recovery.

Neem and Aloe Vera Cooling Mask: Explore neem's antimicrobial powers and aloe vera's cooling and moisturizing benefits. Share a neem and aloe vera mask recipe to soothe inflamed skin and treat acne.

Chamomile and Oatmeal Soothing Mask: Discuss chamomile's anti-inflammatory qualities and oatmeal's mild exfoliation. Provide a recipe for chamomile and oatmeal calming mask to minimize redness and increase skin comfort.

Witch Hazel and Lavender Clarifying Mask: Highlight witch hazel's astringent characteristics and lavender's relaxing benefits. Share a recipe for a witch hazel and lavender clarifying mask to tone the face and minimize acne-related irritation.

Green Tea and Cucumber Refreshing Mask: Explore green tea's antioxidant advantages and cucumber's cooling characteristics. Provide a recipe for a green tea and cucumber refreshing mask to renew the skin and treat acne.

Rosemary and Yogurt Balancing Mask: Discuss Rosemary's antibacterial capabilities and the probiotic advantages of yogurt. Share a recipe for a rosemary and yogurt balancing mask to restore the skin's natural equilibrium.

Lemon and Mint Exfoliating Mask: Highlight lemon's natural exfoliating qualities and mint's pleasant effect. Provide a lemon and mint exfoliation mask recipe to remove dead skin cells and prevent acne outbreaks.

Usage and Consistency Tips: Recommend frequently applying herbal masks for acne-prone skin. Emphasize the value of consistency and patience in monitoring gains over time.

By including these acne-fighting herbal masks in their skincare regimen, users may harness the power of botanicals to treat acne troubles, creating cleaner and healthier skin.

HERBS FOR MENTAL AND EMOTIONAL WELL-BEING: CALMING TEAS AND INFUSIONS

Introduction to Calming Teas: Emphasize herbal teas' relaxing and grounding benefits on mental and emotional well-being. Highlight the significance of herbs in encouraging relaxation and lowering stress.

Chamomile and Lavender Relaxation Blend: Discuss chamomile's soothing characteristics and lavender's stress-relieving benefits. Provide a chamomile and lavender relaxing mix recipe to foster a feeling of peace.

Passionflower and Lemon Balm Stress Relief Infusion: Highlight passionflower's anxiety-reducing capabilities and lemon balm's relaxing benefits. Share a recipe for a passionflower and lemon balm stress relief infusion to alleviate tension and promote relaxation.

Valerian Root and Peppermint Sleepy time Tea: Discuss valerian root's sleep-inducing effects and peppermint's calming characteristics. Provide a recipe for a valerian root and peppermint sleepy time tea to help peaceful sleep and relaxation.

Holy Basil & Rose Petal Harmony Elixir: Explore holy basil's adaptogenic qualities and the relaxing aroma of rose petals. Share a recipe for holy basil and rose petal harmony elixir to balance the mind and raise the soul.

Lemon Verbena and Ginger Digestive Calm Tea: Highlight lemon verbena's relaxing qualities and ginger's digestive advantages. Provide a recipe for a lemon verbena and ginger digestive calm tea to relieve the mind and the stomach.

Linden Flower and Hawthorn Berry Heart-Centered Infusion: Discuss the linden flower's relaxing impact and hawthorn berry's heart-supportive characteristics. Share a recipe for a linden flower and hawthorn berry heart-centered infusion to enhance emotional balance.

Ashwagandha and Licorice Root Stress Adaptogen Tea: Explore ashwagandha's adaptogenic capabilities and licorice root's adrenal support. Provide a recipe for an ashwagandha and licorice root stress adaptogen tea to assist the body in dealing with stress.

Skullcap and Lemon Balm Nervine Tonic: Highlight skullcap's nervine capabilities and lemon balm's relaxing scent. Share a recipe for a skullcap and lemon balm nervine tonic to soothe the nervous system.

Usage and Mindful Brewing Tips: Suggest adopting relaxing teas into regular activities. Encourage attention throughout the brewing process for an increased relaxing experience.

People may nourish their mental and emotional well-being by frequently sipping these peaceful herbal teas, finding moments of quiet in the soft embrace of nature's soothing elixirs.

MEMORY-BOOSTING HERBAL BLENDS

Introduction to Memory-Boosting Blends: Emphasize herbs to promote cognitive function and increase memory. Highlight the synergistic benefits of mixing particular herbs for cognitive well-being.

Ginkgo Biloba and Rosemary Focus Infusion: Discuss Ginkgo Biloba's circulation-boosting capabilities and Rosemary's cognitive-enhancing benefits. Provide a recipe for a Ginkgo biloba and Rosemary focus infusion to improve mental clarity and concentration.

Bacopa Monnieri and Peppermint Brain Boost Tea: Explore Bacopa Monnieri's memory-enhancing abilities and peppermint's revitalizing scent. Share a recipe for a Bacopa monnieri and peppermint brain boost tea to promote mental alertness.

Gotu Kola and Lemon Verbena Clarity Elixir: Highlight Gotu Kola's cognitive assistance and lemon verbena's uplifting characteristics. Provide a recipe for a Gotu kola and lemon verbena clarity elixir to boost mental concentration and awareness.

Turmeric and Cinnamon Cognitive Spice Blend: Discuss turmeric's anti-inflammatory advantages and cinnamon's possible cognitive impacts. Share a recipe for a turmeric and cinnamon cognitive spice combination to add to different recipes for brain health.

Holy Basil and Green Tea Memory Tonic: Explore holy basil's adaptogenic capabilities and green tea's antioxidant advantages. Provide a holy basil and green tea memory tonic recipe to boost general cognitive performance.

Lemon Balm and Sage Memory Infusion: Discuss lemon balm's relaxing impact and sage's memory-boosting reputation. Share a recipe for a lemon balm and sage memory infusion to increase memory retention.

Rhodiola Rosea and Ginger Energizing Elixir: Highlight Rhodiola rosea's adaptogenic benefits and ginger's stimulating characteristics. Provide a recipe for a Rhodiola rosea and ginger revitalizing drink to increase mental endurance and concentration.

Ashwagandha and Cardamom Cognitive Comfort Chai: Explore ashwagandha's stress-reducing properties and cardamom's fragrant features. Share a recipe for an ashwagandha and cardamom cognitive comfort tea to produce a calming and focus-enhancing experience.

Including Brain-Boosting Herbs into Diet: Offer tips on including these memory-boosting herbs into everyday meals. Discuss the relevance of a balanced diet in maintaining general cognitive health.

By routinely savoring these memory-boosting herbal mixes, users may cultivate cognitive function and embrace the advantages of nature's cognitive elixirs for a sharper and more focused mind.

HERBAL SUPPORT FOR STRESS RELIEF

Introduction to Herbal Stress Relief: Emphasize herbs' relaxing and soothing effects in treating stress. Highlight the holistic approach of herbal treatments to enhance mental and emotional well-being.

Chamomile and Lemon Balm Relaxing Infusion: Discuss chamomile's anxiety-reducing benefits and lemon balm's relaxing characteristics. Provide a recipe for a chamomile and lemon balm relaxing infusion to reduce tension and encourage relaxation.

Valerian Root and Lavender Tranquil Tea: Explore valerian root's relaxing impact and lavender's stress-relieving scent. Share a valerian root and lavender calm tea recipe to assist relaxation and ease stress.

Passionflower and Skullcap Nervine Tonic: Highlight passionflower's anxiety-reducing benefits and skullcap's nervine characteristics. Provide a recipe for a passionflower and skullcap nervine tonic to ease the nervous system and encourage calm.

Ashwagandha and Holy Basil Adaptogenic Elixir: Discuss ashwagandha's adaptogenic properties and holy basil's stress-modulating effects. Share a recipe for an ashwagandha and holy basil adaptogenic elixir to assist the body in adapting to stress.

Rhodiola Rosea and Lemon Verbena Energizing Infusion: Explore Rhodiola Rosea's adaptogenic capabilities and lemon verbena's uplifting benefits. Provide a recipe for a Rhodiola rosea and lemon verbena revitalizing infusion to treat stress-induced weariness.

Linden Flower and Hawthorn Berry Heart-Centered Tea: Discuss the linden flower's relaxing impact and hawthorn berry's heart-supportive attributes. Share a recipe for a linden flower and hawthorn berry heart-centered tea to improve emotional balance.

Turmeric and Ginger Anti-Inflammatory Elixir: Highlight turmeric's anti-inflammatory properties and ginger's relaxing influence on the digestive system. Provide a turmeric and ginger anti-inflammatory elixir recipe to relieve stress-related inflammation.

Lemon Balm and Lavender Relaxation Balm: Explore the relaxing qualities of lemon and lavender. Share a recipe for a lemon and lavender relaxation balm to use topically for stress alleviation.

Adopting Stress-Relieving Herbs into Daily Routine: Offer practical tips for adopting these herbs into daily practices. Discuss the value of mindfulness, relaxation methods, and self-care practices in combination with herbal assistance.

By incorporating these stress-relieving herbs into daily routine, people may find refuge in nature's relaxing embrace, cultivating peace and balance amid life's hardships.

HERBAL FIRST AID KIT: CREATING A BASIC HERBAL FIRST AID KIT

Introduction to Herbal First Aid: Emphasize the usefulness of herbs in managing common injuries and disorders. Highlight the value of a herbal first aid kit for natural and holistic treatment.

Calendula Salve for Skin Healing: Discuss calendula's wound-healing and anti-inflammatory qualities. Include a calendula salve to encourage skin healing and ease small wounds, burns, and irritations.

Arnica Gel for Bruise and Muscle Pain: Highlight Arnica's anti-inflammatory and pain-relieving benefits. Include an arnica gel for reducing bruising, swelling, and muscular discomfort.

Lavender Essential Oil for Stress and Minor Burns: Discuss its relaxing effects and capacity to treat burns. Include lavender essential oil for stress reduction and apply directly to mild burns.

Chamomile Tea Bags for Eye Compress: Explore chamomile's anti-inflammatory and calming benefits. Include chamomile tea bags to prepare an eye compress to ease strain and inflammation.

Peppermint Oil for Headache Relief: Highlight peppermint's headache-relieving and cooling effects. Include peppermint oil for topical application to ease headaches and migraines.

Ginger Chews for Nausea: Discuss ginger's anti-nausea and digestive-calming effects. Include ginger chews for managing nausea and motion sickness.

Echinacea Tincture for Immune Support: Explore echinacea's immune-boosting benefits. Include echinacea tincture to help the immune system during mild illnesses.

Activated Charcoal Capsules for Poisoning/Toxin Absorption: Highlight activated charcoal's potential to absorb toxins in the digestive tract. Include activated charcoal tablets for probable poisoning or toxin absorption occurrences.

Cayenne Pepper Powder for Wound Healing: Discuss Cayenne pepper's ability to control bleeding and help heal wounds. Include cayenne pepper powder for its hemostatic qualities in treating small wounds.

Incorporating Holistic methods: Encourage holistic first aid methods, such as deep breathing, relaxation techniques, and awareness. Discuss the necessity of receiving expert medical assistance for major injuries or crises.

By building this simple herbal first aid kit, people may have natural treatments to handle common diseases and accidents, supporting a holistic and herbal approach to personal well-being.

EMERGENCY REMEDIES FOR BURNS AND WOUNDS

Introduction to Emergency Herbal Medicines: Emphasize the rapid and efficient treatment afforded by herbal medicines for burns and wounds. Highlight the necessity of having these solutions readily accessible in emergency circumstances.

Calendula Salve for Burns: Discuss calendula's anti-inflammatory and wound-healing qualities. Include a calendula salve for quick use on burns to soothe and aid healing.

Aloe Vera Gel for Burn Cooling: Highlight aloe vera's cooling and anti-inflammatory benefits. Include aloe vera gel for swiftly cooling and soothing burns, delivering immediate relief.

Lavender Essential Oil for Minor Burns: Discuss lavender's pain-relieving and skin-soothing characteristics. Include lavender essential oil for topical treatment on mild burns to ease pain and reduce inflammation.

Comfrey Poultice for Wounds: Explore comfrey's tissue-regenerating qualities. Prepare a comfrey poultice for wounds to help quickly heal and reduce scarring.

Yarrow Powder for Bleeding Wounds: Highlight Yarrow's hemostatic characteristics that aid in stopping bleeding. Include yarrow powder for quick treatment of bleeding wounds to help with blood clotting.

Chamomile Tea Bags for Compress on Wounds: Discuss chamomile's anti-inflammatory and wound-soothing benefits. Include chamomile tea bags for producing a compress on wounds to decrease swelling and aid healing.

Turmeric Paste for Wound Healing: Explore turmeric's anti-inflammatory and antibacterial effects. Prepare a turmeric paste for wounds to help heal and prevent infection.

Tea Tree Oil for Disinfecting Wounds: Highlight tea tree oil's antibacterial and antiseptic capabilities. Include tea tree oil for cleaning wounds and avoiding infection.

Activated Charcoal Poultice for Toxin Absorption: Discuss activated charcoal's potential to absorb toxins. Prepare an activated charcoal poultice for application to wounds with possible toxin exposure.

Incorporating Emergency Herbal Treatments into First Aid Kit: Provide instructions on creating an emergency herbal kit with these treatments. Emphasize the need to obtain competent medical assistance for serious burns or wounds.

By including these emergency herbal medicines in a first aid pack, people may act rapidly in managing burns and wounds, offering natural comfort and helping the body's healing process in times of need.

NATURAL INSECT REPELLENTS

Introduction to Natural Insect Repellents: Emphasize the usefulness of natural components in repelling insects. Highlight the advantages of avoiding chemical-based repellents.

Lemon Eucalyptus Oil Spray: Discuss lemon eucalyptus oil's proven mosquito-repelling capabilities. Provide a recipe for a lemon eucalyptus oil spray as a natural alternative to chemical repellents.

Citronella Candle Jars: Explore citronella's mosquito-repelling smell. Provide tips on constructing citronella candle jars to create a bug-free outdoor ambiance.

Peppermint and Tea Tree Oil Roller: Highlight peppermint and tea tree oil's insect-repelling capabilities. Provide a peppermint and tea tree oil roller formula for simple and focused application.

Neem Oil Body Lotion: Discuss neem oil's inherent insecticidal capabilities. Provide a neem oil body lotion recipe to nourish the skin while repelling mosquitoes.

Lavender Sachets for Wardrobe: Explore lavender's fragrant characteristics that repel moths and insects. Provide instructions on manufacturing lavender sachets to put in closets and drawers.

Clove and Lemongrass Room Spray: Highlight clove and lemongrass's insect-repelling fragrances. Provide a clove and lemongrass room spray recipe to keep indoor environments bug-free.

Rosemary and Sage Incense Sticks: Discuss Rosemary and Sage's insect-repellent abilities. Provide instructions on creating rosemary and sage incense sticks for outdoor usage.

Cedarwood Repellent Balls: Explore cedarwood's capacity to repel moths and insects. Provide directions on manufacturing cedarwood repellant balls for closets and storage rooms.

Apple Cider Vinegar Mosquito Repellent: Discuss the odor-masking qualities of apple cider vinegar. Provide an apple cider vinegar mosquito repellant spray recipe for indoor and outdoor usage.

Incorporating Natural Repellents into Daily Routine: Offer advice on effortlessly incorporating these natural repellents into daily routines. Emphasize the significance of reapplication for maximum efficiency.

Adding these natural insect repellents into everyday routines allows folks to enjoy the outdoors without harsh chemicals, promoting a bug-free and naturally scented atmosphere.

EXPLORING RARE AND FORGOTTEN REMEDIES: UNCOMMON HERBS WITH POWERFUL BENEFITS

Introduction to Rare Remedies: Emphasize the variety of nature's pharmacy, extending beyond ordinary plants. Highlight the fascination and possibilities of finding uncommon and neglected cures.

Bacopa Monnieri for Cognitive improvement: Discuss Bacopa Monnieri's historical usage for memory improvement. Explore its possible advantages in enhancing cognitive function and mental clarity.

Butterfly Pea Flower for Stress Reduction: Highlight the brilliant blue Butterfly Pea Flower and its historical application in Ayurveda. Discuss its possible stress-reducing and antioxidant qualities.

Rue for Digestive Health: Explore the historical usage of Rue in traditional medicine. Discuss its possible advantages for digestive health and easing gastrointestinal pain.

Blue Tansy for Skin Wellness: Discuss Blue Tansy's unusual blue tint and its skin-soothing effects. Explore its possible advantages in relaxing inflamed skin and increasing overall skin well-being.

Grindelia for Respiratory Support: Highlight Grindelia's historical usage in Native American medicine. Discuss its possible advantages for respiratory support and alleviating breathing issues.

Mugwort for Dream improvement: Explore Mugwort's usage in many civilizations for dream improvement. Discuss its possible advantages in producing vivid dreams and boosting dream memory.

Jiaogulan for Adaptogenic Support: Discuss Jiaogulan's reputation as the "immortality herb" in traditional Chinese medicine. Explore its possible adaptogenic characteristics and advantages for general well-being.

Wood Betony for Headache Relief: Highlight Wood Betony's historical usage in European herbalism. Discuss its possible advantages in alleviating headaches and stress.

Galangal for Digestive Aid: Discuss Galangal's similarities to ginger and its usage in traditional medicine. Explore its possible advantages in assisting digestion and relieving gastrointestinal disorders.

Adopting Uncommon Herbs into Daily Wellness: Suggest adopting these uncommon herbs into daily routines. Emphasize the necessity of studying and speaking with healthcare experts before utilizing unusual cures.

By researching these unusual herbs, people may unleash the potential advantages of nature's lesser-known gems, improving their health journey with various cures.

TRADITIONAL REMEDIES FROM INDIGENOUS CULTURES

Introduction to Indigenous Healing Practices: Emphasize the fundamental link between indigenous cultures and the healing power of nature. Highlight the comprehensive approach of traditional treatments in improving bodily and spiritual well-being.

Willow Bark Tea for Pain Management (Native American): Discuss the usage of willow bark by Native American cultures for pain management. Explore the analgesic and anti-inflammatory benefits of willow bark tea.

Kava Kava for Relaxation (Pacific Islands): Highlight the traditional usage of kava kava in Pacific Island cultures for relaxation. Discuss its soothing effects on the nervous system and its importance in social and ceremonial situations.

Eucalyptus Steam Inhalation (Aboriginal Australian): Discuss the Australian usage of eucalyptus for respiratory wellness. Explore the technique of steam inhalation using eucalyptus leaves to ease congestion and respiratory difficulties.

Maca Root for vigor (Andean tribes): Explore the historical usage of maca root by Andean tribes for energy and vigor. Discuss its adaptogenic qualities and possible advantages in improving endurance.

Ashwagandha for Stress Relief (Ayurveda - India): Discuss the traditional Ayurvedic usage of ashwagandha for stress and anxiety. Explore its adaptogenic capabilities and its function in boosting general well-being.

Turmeric Golden Milk (Ayurveda - India): Highlight the Ayurvedic usage of turmeric in the renowned Golden Milk. Discuss the anti-inflammatory and immune-boosting benefits of turmeric.

Ginseng Tonic for Energy (Traditional Chinese Medicine): Discuss the traditional usage of Ginseng in Chinese medicine for energy and vigor. Explore its adaptogenic properties and possible advantages for physical endurance.

Coca Leaf Chewing (Andean Cultures): Highlight the cultural importance of coca leaf chewing in Andean nations. Discuss its historical usage for altitude sickness, vitality, and mental clarity.

Pine Needle Tea (numerous Indigenous societies): Discuss the extensive usage of pine needle tea in numerous indigenous societies. Explore its possible health advantages, including vitamin C content and immunological support.

Honoring and Preserving Indigenous Wisdom: Emphasize the significance of honoring indigenous knowledge and customs. Discuss the necessity for ethical and sustainable procedures while acquiring traditional treatments.

By embracing the knowledge of indigenous cultures, people may receive insights into time-tested cures that recognize the connection between environment and human well-being. It is vital to approach and embrace these practices with cultural awareness and genuine respect for the communities that have maintained these traditions for centuries.

REDISCOVERING LOST HEALING PLANTS

Introduction to Lost Healing Plants: Emphasize the abundance of healing knowledge that past societies held. Highlight the significance of finding and protecting neglected therapeutic plants.

Spikenard for Relaxation and Sleep: Discuss the historical usage of spikenard in old herbal systems. Explore its possible advantages in generating relaxation and enhancing sleep quality.

Sweet Annie for Digestive Health: Highlight the historical usage of sweet Annie in traditional medicine. Discuss its possible advantages in maintaining digestive health and easing gastrointestinal pain.

Mullein for Respiratory Support: Discuss the historical usage of mullein in different herbal systems. Explore its potential advantages in providing respiratory support and alleviating breathing issues.

Elecampane for Immune Boost: Highlight the historical usage of elecampane in herbal treatments. Discuss its possible advantages in strengthening the immune system and managing respiratory disorders.

Horehound for Cough Relief: Discuss the historical usage of horehound for respiratory illnesses. Explore its possible advantages in easing coughs and enhancing respiratory health.

Mandrake for Pain Management: Highlight the historical usage of mandrake in ancient medicine. Discuss its possible advantages in treating pain and discomfort.

Beth Root for Women's Health: Discuss the historical usage of Beth Root in traditional medicine. Explore its potential advantages in supporting women's health, especially during menstruation.

Tansy for Skin Conditions: Highlight the historical usage of tansy in herbal medicines. Discuss its potential advantages in managing skin issues and boosting skin wellbeing.

Mayapple for Digestive Issues: Discuss the historical usage of mayapple in Native American traditional medicine. Explore its potential advantages in managing digestive disorders and boosting gut health.

Restoring Lost knowledge: Emphasize the necessity of maintaining and restoring traditional herbal knowledge. Discuss the importance of current science in verifying the effectiveness of these forgotten healing herbs.

By rediscovering and combining these ancient healing plants into modern practices, people may tap into the vast pool of traditional knowledge, exploring natural treatments that have endured the test of time. Treating these plants with respect is vital, considering ethical harvesting procedures and engaging with herbal specialists when studying their potential benefits.

CULTIVATING YOUR HERBAL GARDEN: PLANNING AND DESIGNING A MEDICINAL GARDEN

Introduction to Medicinal Gardens: Emphasize the delight of growing a garden that beautifies and supplies therapeutic herbs. Highlight the therapeutic advantages of being near nature.

Choosing the Right Site: Discuss the significance of sunshine, soil quality, and drainage in finding the optimal garden site. Consider variables like accessibility and closeness to water sources.

Selecting Therapeutic Plants: Identify certain plants based on their therapeutic characteristics and compatibility with your location. Consider perennial and annual herbs for a diversified and year-round garden.

Companion Planting for Health: Explore companion planting ideas for pest control and mutual benefit. Pair herbs that compliment one other's growth and promote overall garden health.

Creating routes and Seating Areas: Design routes for simple access and upkeep. Integrate sitting places to enjoy the therapeutic aura of the medicinal garden

Organizing Plant Beds: Plan the arrangement of plant beds for visual appeal and efficient upkeep. Consider clustering plants with comparable water and sunshine needs.

Incorporating Water Elements: Integrate water elements like a small pond or fountain for aesthetic and relaxing benefits. Consider water-loving plants in the vicinity of water features.

Adding Decorative pieces: Enhance the garden's visual appeal with decorative pieces like garden art or sculptures. Ensure these features complement the natural atmosphere of the medicinal garden.

Implementing Sustainable methods: Emphasize organic and sustainable gardening methods. Consider composting, rainwater gathering, and natural pest control options.

Designing a Healing Corner: Create a designated spot for mindfulness and relaxation within the garden. Include comfy chairs, fragrant plants, and calming colors for a therapeutic environment.

Educational Signage and Labels: Install labels and signage for each plant, offering educational information. Share facts about the therapeutic characteristics and historical applications of the cultivated plants.

Regular Maintenance and Care: Develop a watering, trimming, and harvesting regimen. Encourage attention throughout maintenance tasks for a soothing gardening experience.

Gathering and Preserving Herbs: Educate on the right time and practices for gathering therapeutic herbs. Provide tips on drying and storing herbs for future use.

By carefully planning and building a therapeutic garden, people may create a harmonious setting that feeds the body and rejuvenates the mind and spirit. This purposeful cultivation develops a closer connection to nature and the therapeutic powers of herbs.

GROWING AND HARVESTING HERBS

Selecting the Right Herbs: Choose herbs according to climate, soil conditions, and available space. Consider both culinary and medicinal herbs to maximize the variety of your garden.

Creating a Suitable Herb Garden: Designate a well-drained location with adequate sunshine for best herb growth. Depending on available space, utilize containers, raised beds, or standard garden beds.

Providing Proper Soil and Nutrients: Ensure well-draining soil filled with compost or organic debris. Consider soil testing to discover and manage individual nutritional demands for various plants.

Watering Practices: Develop a regular watering plan, considering the water needs of various herbs. Water at the base of the plants to prevent fungal concerns and encourage healthy root growth.

Companion Planting: Implement companion planting to increase herb growth and discourage pests. Pair herbs that mutually benefit each other, such as basil and tomatoes.

Pruning and Trimming: Regularly prune herbs to promote bushier growth and avoid legginess. Harvest or trim herbs selectively to maintain ongoing growth throughout the growing season.

Managing Pests Naturally: Use natural pest management strategies like companion planting and introducing helpful insects. Regularly monitor plants for symptoms of pests and take quick action.

Harvesting Timing and Techniques: Harvest herbs when they have achieved their optimum taste or medicinal efficacy. Utilize clean and sharp scissors or pruning shears to prevent injuring the plant.

Drying Herbs for Preservation: Choose the correct technique for drying herbs, such as air drying, dehydrating, or oven drying. Ensure appropriate ventilation and eliminate moisture to prevent mold throughout the drying process.

Freezing and Storing Fresh Herbs: Consider freezing herbs to retain freshness and taste. Store dried or frozen herbs in sealed containers away from light and heat.

Seed Saving: Learn about seed-saving practices to build a sustainable herb garden. Allow some plants to grow to seed, collect, and store them for future plantings.

Continuous Learning and Experimentation: Stay interested and continue learning about the special demands of various herbs. Experiment with various types and growth strategies to improve your herb garden.

Sharing and Community Involvement: Share excess herbs with neighbors or local community members. Engage in herb-related community activities or gardening organizations for collective knowledge.

By planting and harvesting herbs with care and attention, folks may enjoy the freshness of homegrown tastes and harness the therapeutic advantages of various herb gardens. It becomes a path of ongoing learning, exploration, and a profound connection to the natural world.

TIPS FOR SUSTAINABLE HERBAL GARDENING

Native Plant Selection: Opt for native herbs well-adapted to your local ecology. Native plants generally demand fewer resources and maintain local biodiversity.

Water Conservation: Implement effective watering strategies, such as drip irrigation or soaker hoses. Collect rainwater for watering plants, decreasing dependency on municipal water sources.

Organic Soil Enrichment: Use organic mulch and compost to boost soil fertility. Avoid synthetic fertilizers and pesticides to create a healthy ecology.

Companion Planting: Employ companion planting to naturally prevent pests and boost development. Integrate herbs that complement one other's growth patterns and nutritional demands.

Polyculture Gardening: Embrace polyculture by cultivating various herbs in the same location. This replicates natural ecosystems, encouraging resilience and lowering the danger of pests and illnesses.

Natural Pest Control: Encourage beneficial insects like ladybugs and predatory beetles. Introduce companion plants that resist common herb pests.

Chemical-Free Weed Management: Utilize hand weeding, mulching, or cover cropping to manage weeds. Avoid synthetic herbicides that may affect soil health and beneficial organisms.

Seed Saving and Exchange: Engage in seed-saving methods to enhance biodiversity and sustainability. Participate in seed exchanges with local gardeners to diversify your herbal garden.

Permaculture concepts: Apply permaculture concepts such as planning for many uses and leveraging natural patterns. Create guilds of plants that work together synergistically.

Habitat Creation: Incorporate elements like bird baths, bug motels, or native plant borders to attract beneficial species. Enhance the overall ecological health of your garden.

Reuse and Recycle: Repurpose materials for garden structures and containers. Reuse kitchen leftovers and yard trash for composting, completing the loop on organic matter.

Mindful Harvesting: Harvest herbs mindfully, enabling plants to regrow and flourish. Avoid overharvesting and consider the long-term health of your herbal garden.

Educational Outreach: Share sustainable gardening methods with your community. Educate people on the value of biodiversity and the advantages of herbal gardening.

By combining these sustainable techniques, herbal gardening becomes a regenerative and nourishing enterprise, generating a resilient ecosystem that benefits both the environment and the individuals growing the garden.

ETHICAL CONSIDERATIONS IN HERBAL MEDICINE: RESPONSIBLE FORAGING PRACTICES

Respect for Ecosystems: Harvest herbs in a manner that minimizes harm to local ecosystems. Avoid overharvesting and be careful of the balance within the natural ecosystem.

Identify and Learn: Properly identify herbs before harvesting to avoid unintentionally collecting endangered or protected species. Continuously educate oneself on sustainable foraging tactics.

Harvesting Ethics: Harvest just what you need, keeping the bulk of the plant intact to encourage its growth and reproduction. Consider the plant's life cycle and prevent harvesting from populations in danger.

Location Awareness: Respect private property rights and ask permission before foraging on private territory. Be careful of local rules regulating foraging in public locations.

Avoiding Threatened Species: Refrain from collecting endangered, rare, or fragile plants. Consult local conservation groups or plant databases to identify a plant's conservation status.

Cultivate Rather Than Harvest: Consider producing herbs in a garden rather than foraging from the wild when available. This helps lessen the strain on wild species and supports sustainable practices.

Mindful Foraging Ethics: Practice awareness when foraging, minimizing harm to nearby species and plant populations. Leave no trace by avoiding harm to the environment and reducing disruptions.

Conservation Efforts: Support conservation programs that maintain and preserve native plant species. Contribute to or participate in local habitat restoration efforts.

Ethical Wildcrafting: Engage in ethical wildcrafting, which incorporates sustainable harvesting procedures and a dedication to environmental management. Share information and encourage responsible foraging within your community.

Seasonal Awareness: Be aware of the seasons and the life cycles of plants. Harvest herbs at the proper periods to maintain their vigor and resistance.

Documentation and Record-Keeping: Maintain records on foraging areas, techniques, and the influence on plant populations. This material may serve as a great resource for ethical foraging in the future.

Cultural Sensitivity: Respect the cultural relevance of plants to indigenous cultures. Understand and adhere to any cultural standards or prohibitions linked to foraging.

By embracing these ethical principles, people may enjoy the advantages of herbal therapy while actively contributing to preserving biodiversity and managing natural resources. Responsible foraging procedures guarantee that picking herbs is connected with conservation values and environmental respect.

CONSERVATION OF MEDICINAL PLANTS

Identification and Assessment: Conduct extensive evaluations to identify medicinal plant species in their native settings. Evaluate each species' ecological state and population health to evaluate conservation requirements.

Habitat Protection: Implement steps to maintain and preserve the natural habitats of medicinal plants. Establish and manage protected areas, reserves, or botanical sanctuaries to conserve key ecosystems.

Community Engagement: Involve local communities in conservation activities, honoring their traditional wisdom. Collaborate with indigenous and local populations to create sustainable harvesting techniques and participate in the benefits of conservation.

Cultivation and Propagation: Encourage the cultivation of medicinal plants using sustainable agricultural techniques. Promote the proliferation of endangered species in botanical gardens or controlled habitats.

Study and Monitoring: Conduct continuing studies to understand plant species' ecology, biology, and therapeutic characteristics.

Implement monitoring procedures to observe population changes and assess the efficacy of conservation efforts.

Legal safeguards: Advocate for and support legal safeguards for endangered medicinal plants. Work towards enforcing current regulations controlling these plants' collection, trading, and transportation.

Ethical Wildcrafting rules: Establish and promote ethical wildcrafting rules for sustainable harvesting. Educate herbalists, foragers, and the general public on ethical harvesting procedures.

Collaboration with Stakeholders: Collaborate with governmental agencies, NGOs, and research institutions to pool resources and expertise. Foster relationships that solve conservation concerns on a bigger scale.

Seed Banks and Ex Situ Conservation: Establish seed banks to retain genetic material of endangered medicinal plants. Explore ex-situ conservation strategies, such as cultivating plants outside their native environment under controlled settings.

Education and Awareness: Raise awareness about the necessity of medicinal plant conservation. Educate the public, politicians, and stakeholders on the importance of these plants in traditional medicine and global health.

Incentives for Sustainable Techniques: Incentivizes communities and individuals to adopt sustainable techniques in producing and collecting medicinal plants. Develop certification systems that reward adherence to conservation principles.

Climate Change Considerations: Factor in the possible implications of climate change on medicinal plant ecosystems. Develop adaptive techniques to guarantee the resilience of plant populations under changing environmental circumstances.

Restoration Initiatives: Support restoration programs to repair damaged ecosystems and reestablish therapeutic plant species. Engage local communities in habitat restoration operations to boost ecological health.

By taking a holistic approach to medicinal plant conservation, we can secure the preservation of these vital resources for future generations while supporting sustainable practices that benefit both ecosystems and human health.

SUPPORTING LOCAL HERBAL COMMUNITIES

Community cooperation: Foster cooperation amongst local herbalists, producers, and practitioners. Create forums for exchanging information, experiences, and traditional wisdom within the community.

Herbal Education Programs: Establish educational programs to empower community people with herbal knowledge. Conduct workshops, seminars, and training sessions on sustainable herbal practices.

Cultivating Herbal Gardens: Encourage the creation of communal herbal gardens. Provide resources and assistance for villagers to produce and share medicinal plants collaboratively.

Local Herb Markets: Facilitate local herb markets or fairs to promote and sell herbal items. Promote economic possibilities for local herbalists and producers.

Traditional Medicine Clinics: Support the creation of traditional medicine clinics within the community. Provide resources for practitioners to give inexpensive or free herbal consultations.

Access to Resources: Ensure local herbalists access excellent seeds, sustainable harvesting procedures, and ethical sourcing. Collaborate with organizations to give resources for cultivation and preservation.

Fair Trade Practices: Advocate for fair trade practices in the herbal sector. Ensure that local herbal communities get appropriate compensation for their expertise and products.

Cultural Preservation: Support programs that conserve and appreciate the cultural history of herbal traditions. Document and disseminate local tales, customs, and rituals relating to herbal medicine.

Community Apothecaries: Establish community apothecaries where herbal items are manufactured and shared. Promote the sharing of remedies and information among community members.

Collaboration with Indigenous Communities: Collaborate with indigenous communities to learn from and respect their traditional herbal methods. Support projects that empower indigenous herbalists and preserve their unique expertise.

Sustainable gathering standards: Develop and distribute standards for sustainable gathering of native medicinal plants. Educate community members on safe foraging techniques to guarantee long-term supply.

Networking Platforms: Create networking platforms or organizations for local herbalists to connect and assist one other.

Facilitate communication and the sharing of resources within the herbal community.

Government Advocacy: Support government policies that recognize and safeguard traditional herbal practices. Encourage the integration of herbal medicine into local healthcare systems.

By supporting local herbal communities, we contribute to people's well-being and help conserve and develop the rich tapestry of herbal traditions that constitute an intrinsic part of cultural identity and health practices.

PLANT IDENTIFICATION GUIDE

A:

Aloe Vera (Aloe barbadensis miller):

Succulent with thick, meaty leaves.

The gel within leaves is used for burns and skin irritations.

B:

Bacopa Monnieri (Bacopa):

Creeping plant with tiny, oblong leaves.

Used for cognitive boosting and memory assistance.

Beth Root (Trillium erectum):

Perennial plant with a triad of leaves and a center bloom.

Traditional usage in women's health.

Blue Tansy (Tanacetum annuum):

Herb with tiny, daisy-like blue blooms.

Used for skin well-being and relaxing characteristics.

Butterfly Pea Flower (Clitoria ternatea):

Climbing vine with vivid blue blossoms.

Traditionally used for stress alleviation.

C:

Calendula (Calendula officinalis):

Bright orange or yellow blossoms.

Used in salves for burns and skin disorders.

Chamomile (Matricaria chamomilla):

Daisy-like blossoms with a pleasant smell.

Used for relaxing drinks and compresses.

Coca Leaf (Erythroxylum coca):

Evergreen shrub with oval leaves.

Traditionally chewed for energy and altitude sickness.

Comfrey (Symphytum officinale):

Herb with hairy leaves and bell-shaped blooms.

Used in poultices for wound healing.

E:

Elecampane (Inula helenium):

Tall herb with yellow blooms.

Used for immune support and respiratory disorders.

Eucalyptus (Eucalyptus spp.):

Tall evergreen tree with fragrant leaves.

Leaves are used in steam inhalation for respiratory health.

G:

Galangal (Alpinia galanga):

Rhizomatous plant with fragrant roots.

Used for digestive assistance in traditional medicine.

Grindelia (Grindelia spp.):

Herb with yellow blooms and aromatic leaves.

Used for respiratory assistance.

H:

Horehound (Marrubium vulgare):

Gray-green leaves with white fuzzy hairs.

Used for cough alleviation in herbal medicines.

J:

Jiaogulan (Gynostemma pentaphyllum):

Climbing vine with serrated leaves.

Known as the "immortality herb" in traditional Chinese medicine.

L:

Lavender (Lavandula angustifolia):

Fragrant plant with spike-like blooms.

Essential oil is used for burns and relaxation.

Lemon Balm (Melissa officinalis):

Fragrant plant with lemon-scented leaves.

Used in relaxing teas and infusions.

Lungwort (Pulmonaria officinalis):

Herb with speckled leaves.

Historically used for respiratory difficulties.

M:

Maca Root (Lepidium meyenii):

Radish-like root vegetable.

Used for vitality and energy support.

Mandrake (Mandragora officinarum):

Herbaceous plant with a rosette of leaves.

Historically used for pain management.

Mayapple (Podophyllum peltatum):

Herb with huge, umbrella-like leaves.

Used in Native American medicine for intestinal disorders.

Memory-Boosting Herbal Blends:

Blends of herbs include ginkgo, rosemary, and gotu kola.

Used for cognitive improvement.

Mugwort (Artemisia vulgaris):

Herb with strongly lobed leaves.

Traditionally used for dream enhancing.

Mullein (Verbascum thapsus):

Tall plant with fuzzy leaves.

Used for respiratory assistance.

N:

Neem (Azadirachta indica): Evergreen tree with pinnate leaves.

Oil is extracted for its antimicrobial effects.

P:

Peppermint (Mentha × Piperita):

Aromatic herb with serrated leaves.

Used for digestive assistance and soothing teas.

Pine (Pinus spp.):

Evergreen tree with needle-like leaves.

Needles are used for pine needle tea.

R:

Rue (Ruta graveolens):

Herb with bluish-green leaves.

Used for intestinal health in traditional medicine.

S:

Spikenard (Nardostachys jatamansi):

Herb with rhizomes and fragrant roots.

Used for relaxation and sleep support.

Sweet Annie (Artemisia annua):

Herb with fern-like leaves.

Used for intestinal health.

T:

Tansy (Tanacetum vulgare):

Herb with yellow button-like blooms.

Used for skin problems.

Tea Tree (Melaleuca alternifolia):

Small tree with needle-like leaves.

Essential oil used for cleaning wounds.

Turmeric (Curcuma longa):

Herbaceous plant with rhizomes.

It is used in golden milk for its anti-inflammatory effects.

U:

Uncommon Herbs with Powerful Benefits:

Various unusual plants include spikenard, butterfly pea blossom, and more.

Each has distinct benefits for comprehensive well-being.

W:

Willow (Salix spp.):

Deciduous tree with thin leaves.

The bark is used for pain alleviation.

Wood Betony (Stachys officinalis):

Herb with prickly blooms.

Used traditionally for headache alleviation.

Y:

Yarrow (Achillea millefolium):

Herb with feathery leaves and umbrella-like blooms.

Used for bleeding wounds.

This guide gives a starting point for identifying therapeutic plants based on their primary properties. Always use care and, when in doubt, check with an expert herbalist or botanist for precise plant identification.

CONCLUSION

In closing, in this herbal compendium, we start on a journey that celebrates the complex dance between humans and the healing richness of nature. From the soothing touch of Aloe Vera to the stimulating scent of Ginseng, each article in this book is a monument to the deep relationship humans have with plant life.

As we go into the chapters investigating cures for burns, respiratory problems, and skin disorders, we discover the ageless knowledge buried in ancient herbal techniques. The alphabetically structured index acts as a doorway, enabling readers to browse easily across the enormous terrain of herbal medicines, finding peace in nature's solutions.

From the conscientious concerns of sustainable gardening to the ethical nuances of responsible foraging, this book attempts to build a healthy connection between people and the environment. Embracing ancient knowledge and indigenous methods, we appreciate the roots of herbal wisdom.

The chapters on recovering forgotten healing plants and researching unusual cures call us to become stewards of biodiversity, maintaining and perpetuating the rich tapestry of natural medicines for centuries to come. The development of herbal gardens, whether in communal places or personal sanctuaries, becomes a canvas onto which we paint the colors of sustainability, awareness, and well-being.

The dedication to ethical standards, fair trade, and community development reinforces the notion that herbal medicine is a transaction and a reciprocal interaction between persons and the environment. It is a recognition of the connectivity that characterizes holistic health and the complicated fabric of life.

In supporting local herbal communities, we honor the guardians of traditional knowledge, acknowledging their vital role in maintaining cultural heritage. The necessity of conservation rings loudly, calling us to become champions for preserving medicinal plants and their environments.

As we say farewell to these pages, let us take on the knowledge taught by the medicines, the ethical considerations, and the cultivation methods. May we become ambassadors of herbal health, caring for our gardens, encouraging sustainable practices, and accepting the deep knowledge that nature lovingly bestows upon us. In conclusion, may this book be a companion on your journey—a guide that whispers the earth's secrets, reminding us that we discover the genuine essence of well-being in the delicate balance between healer and healed. May your discovery of herbal treatments be a source of inspiration, empowerment, and a closer connection to the natural world.